MW01295504

Essential Oils

The Young Living Book Guide of Natural Remedies for Beginners for Pets, For Dogs

LELA GIBSON

LELA GIBSON

Copyright © 2017 Lela Gibson

All rights reserved.

LELA GIBSON

CONTENTS

ESSENTIAL OILS

Introduction

I want to thank you and congratulate you for buying the book, "Essential Oils: The Young Living Book Guide of Natural Remedies for Beginners for Pets, For Dogs".

This book has lots of actionable information on how to use essential oils on pets.

Since you are reading this, you love your pet and because you know the benefits of essential oils, you want your pet to enjoy the benefits of essential oils just as you do. Essential oils are important to us for many reasons; they are also important to pets. For pets, most of these reasons are no different.

Whether you want to improve your dog's digestive function, skin, respiration, immune support for seasonal and environmental health or even for purposes of repelling insects, with the essential oils we are going to talk about today, you can do that safely and naturally.

More specifically, we will discuss the right types of essential oils, the proper application process, and something about the essential oils issues that have made it difficult for cautious folks to use these oils on their pets.

First, there are different forms of essential oils available today and animals metabolize and react differently to each of them. This alone has become a major concern. It is thus important that we all understand things such as the species-specific differences before using the essential oils.

In addition, many vets often observe a big problem in their clinics: issues related to overusing of essential oils—people discover essential oils and wildly start diffusing them into their homes and end up creating unintentional overdoses for their pets—we shall discuss and clarify this issue.

The purpose of this book is to help you avert such issues and help you know how best to use natural essential oils to increase the appetite, reduce fatigue, boost the immune system, remove anxiety, and manage many other problems that hinder your pet's wellbeing.

Thanks again for buying this book. I hope you enjoy it!

Before we start discussing how to use essential oils on pets, let's start by understanding essential oils.

Understanding Essential Oils

What are essential oils, really?

The words "essential oil" comes from the word "quintessential oil," a word stemming from an archaic idea that matter consists of four main elements that include air, water, earth, and fire. Quintessence was then regarded as the fifth element and was considered life force or spirit. Since part of the process of making essential oils involve distillation and evaporation, essential oils were considered the process of removing the spirit part from a plant (perhaps no wonder we use the term spirits to describe different distilled alcoholic beverages like eau de vie, whiskey, and brandy).

Today, we know that essential oils are far from being spirit; they are physical in nature and consist of complex chemical mixtures. An essential oil contains the 'essential' chemical and aromatic properties of the plant from which it comes. These chemical compounds are important because they directly affect the normal functioning of the body to bring about desirable effects.

For instance, we have Terpenes that inhibit the accumulation of toxins and discharge them from kidneys and liver, and Aldehydes that mainly counter infections, offer sedative effects, and calm the body upon inhalation of essential oil aromas that have these properties. So how exactly do essential oils achieve all that? Let's discuss that next:

How Essential Oils Interact With Bodily Systems

Essential oils usually enter the body through two routes: through the skin and through the nose. Let us look at how they work through each.

Through The Nose (Inhalation)

When you smell essential oils, the small hairs in the nostrils pick up the particles. The particles then quickly absorb into the mucous lining before the aroma finally reaches the brain's 'smell center' called the olfactory bulb.

This center changes the aroma into some sort of a neural code conveyed across to the limbic system or the 'emotional center' and further to the hippocampus or the temporary memory center and the hypothalamus or long-term memory center. The information then passes on to the pituitary gland or the 'master gland' and other endocrine glands, and the body secretes 'feel good' hormones to reinstate hormonal balance.

Just to put it straight, it goes like this: **the nose>smell center>temporary memory>permanent memory>master gland>endocrine system.**

This simple reaction makes the brain create connection between particular smells, emotions, and memories that it responds to in a predictable manner.

For instance, your coworker professes his love for you and gives you beautiful roses. Your brain directly associates the smell with a romantic emotion and for a long period (in future), the fragrance makes you feel nostalgic and romantic. For you and your pet, inhalation is particularly a great way to relieve emotional issues such as anxiety, stress, and depression.

Through The Skin (Topical Application)

As mentioned earlier, essential oils usually undergo a distillation process to produce the smallest and finest molecules. These molecules can penetrate the epidermis (outer skin layer) and the smaller they are, the faster the absorption rate. The molecules also penetrate through the dermis (inner skin layers) and into the bloodstream through capillaries from where they go to different sections of the body.

The oil molecules have specific biochemical features that help them bind to cell receptors in the organ of target and work as a tonic for the same. As the oils travel in the body, they function to detoxify and revitalize the organs involved in drainage and metabolism (lymphatic network, kidney, and liver).

In short, the process goes like this: **epidermis>dermis>capillaries>bloodstream>organs targeted>cell receptors>metabolized and excreted.**

This method of essential oil application is more holistic since it seeks to even up all body systems.

The good news is that essential oils are natural compounds. This means they do not deposit themselves in the cells and the body removes them through sweat, exhalation, and urine within a day. So how exactly can you use essential oils on pets? That's what we will discuss next.

Essential Oils and Pets

Now that you know what essential oils are and how they work, we can now talk about how they affect pets, the best types of essential oils to use on your pets, and how to apply them. Since pets are many, our primary focus shall be cats and dogs to represent other pets since these two are the most common types of pets.

Pets and Essential Oils: The Benefits

Based on the numerous natural compounds they contain, essential oils come with numerous benefits, most of which animals can enjoy too. In general, the key/most noted benefits for pets include the following:

1.   They naturally calm pets. If your dog is fearful, anxious, hyperactive, or agitated, using the right essential oils will take care of that for him/her.

2.   Tick and flea control. The essential oils are also helpful in repelling parasites such as ticks and fleas even though they do not really kill them.

3.   Most pets tend to adopt bad odors that can be very irritating. The good thing is that essential oils are not just medicinal: they can also give a fresh, great fragrance to your pet.

4.   If your pet has dry, itchy skin, some essential oils can take care of that to provide relief and better skin. Many people using essential oils for animal skin therapy have offered positive reports in regards to their benefit in remedying stings, insect bites, and skin rashes.

5.   Essential oils have antiseptic qualities ideal for cleaning a pet's bedding.

6.   Owing to their inhalant properties, essential oils are important in respiratory therapy; this means the right essential oil can help fight respiratory problems such as like bronchitis and sinus infections.

What You Need To Know Before Starting Application

Essential oils are generally safe to use around many kinds of pets that can benefit from their use in multiple ways. If your pet is a large herbivores animal such as alpacas, cattle, llamas, or even goats and sheep, you can apply the essential oils topically directly to the concerning area even without diluting them or along the spine just as you would apply them to yourself. When dealing with smaller animals such as dogs and cats, you should exercise more care.

It is actually quite interesting how many pet owners are comfortable with diffusing commercial, chemical-laced air fresheners in almost every room in their houses without considering the possibility of causing harm, but get overly worried about how use of essential oils shall harm their pets. This is a good thing.

We should all be cautious about the 'small things' when we have pets around us. We should also appreciate that like humans, individual animals have their own sensitivities, preferences, and dislikes. Therefore, always closely observe your pet's behavior to establish a baseline, and with that, you will notice any behavioral change when you start using a particular essential oil.

If your pet continues behaving normally, everything is okay; however, if you observe the opposite, the pet may be sensitive to the oil. Animals are always good at communicating their feelings.

Cats

Cats naturally lack an important enzyme in their liver that is necessary in the metabolism of many sorts of things. This normally makes the cats vulnerable to all sorts of toxicity including plant, lead, zinc, pesticides, caffeine (methylxanthines), and NSAIDS (such as ibuprofen, Tylenol, and aspirin).

Try as much as possible to avoid using essential oils high in ketones and phenols especially when using the topical application method. Such essential oils include cinnamon, basil, melaleuca, birch, nutmeg, clove, thyme, peppermint, oregano, rosemary, wintergreen, fennel, and spearmint. Cats are also sensitive to oils containing d-limonene such as lemon, grape fruit, orange, tangerine, bergamot, dill, lime, and tangerine.

You should note that the use of essential oils on cats is not something you should favor because of cats' high sensitivity to many of the ingredients in commonly used essential oils. This means when using essential oils on your pet cat, you have to take extra caution and except in instances where you want to treat particular ailments, you should avoid them unless you are using them under the supervision of a veterinarian, and when diluted.

If applied to the cat's skin or ingested, the oils can damage the skin, or even induce seizures. If your cat accidentally ingests an essential oil, get your cat to the veterinarian immediately.

Dogs

Firstly, compared to humans, dogs are a tad more sensitive to essential oils. Therefore, make sure you always dilute essential oils before use on your dog even if the mode of application is inhalation. This is very important to note because when it comes to inhaling essential oils, most people ignore dilution.

Using diluted essential oils for inhalation, you can address most issues dogs usually experience. There are, however, some issues you can address with topical use, as you will soon learn.

Secondly, always remember to use essential oils with your dog to address a concern, and never to prevent a health issue. For instance, some people will have their dogs inhale digestive essential oils after the dogs have eaten as a way to prevent any digestive problem even when the dog has not shown signs of having such a problem. DO NOT DO THIS!

Never add essential oils to your dog's food or drinking water.

In addition, if you have a puppy whose age is under 10 weeks, do not use essential oils on such a pup; instead, use hydrosols.

Finally, when offering essential oils to your dog, first try pre-selecting 3-5 essential oils from the 'safe list' you think are most effective for the problem that requires attention. Usually, a number of essential oils can be beneficial, and letting your dog select which one in particular will make sure you do not go wrong.

Important: Dilute All Essential Oils

As a general rule for all pets, (and especially cats), always dilute the essential oils with a high grade pure vegetable oil— fractionated coconut oil is one of the best. For cats and other smaller animals, use the ration 50:1 –this means 50 drops of dilution oil to 1 drop of essential oil. You can follow this rule in instances when a specific remedy does not specify the ration.

Next, we will discuss how to use essential oils on common pets.

Using Essential Oils with Common Pets

As you know, not all essential oils are safe and not all safe essential oils are applicable to all animals. Moreover, in some instances, the mode of application for different animals is not the same. Let us discuss that in detail:

Dogs: Selecting Safe/The Best Essential Oils for Dogs

For dogs, you should only go for the following essential oils:

Carrot Seed (Daucus carota)

Its properties include the following:

It is tonic, anti-inflammatory, and has moderate antibacterial effects. This oil is good for dry, flaky, and sensitive skin prone to infection. It can revitalize and trigger tissue regeneration; it is thus effective for healing of scars.

Cedarwood (Juniperus virginiana)

This is a great essential oil to use for tonic, antiseptic, and circulation stimulation purposes. It is great for coat and skin conditioning, and dermatitis of all sorts. It is also a great flea repellant.

Chamomile, German (Matricaria recutita)

Chamomile essential oil is a good non-toxic, anti-inflammatory, and very gentle essential oil that is also great for skin irritations, burns, and allergic reactions.

Chamomile, Roman (Chamaemelum nobile)

This essential oil is special for its analgesic, antispasmodic, and nerve calming properties and thus great for calming the central nervous system and very effective for cramps relief, teething pain, and muscle pains. If you own a dog, you should always have this essential oil in close proximity.

Clary Sage (Salvia sclarea)

This essential oil is popular for its effectiveness in sedating the central nervous system thanks to its nerve-calming properties. It is very gentle when you dilute it well and use it in small amounts. However, avoid using it on pregnant dogs.

Eucalyptus Radiata (Eucalyptus radiata)

This is another anti-inflammatory, antiviral, and an expectorant essential oil that is a good choice for relieving chest congestion. You should avoid using it with puppies and small dogs.

Geranium (Pelargonium x asperum)

The Geranium essential oil is mainly antifungal in nature. It is great for fungal ear infections, skin irritations, and is very effective in repelling ticks. It is also gentle and safer to use.

Ginger (Zingiber officinale)

This essential oil is also non-irritating, non-toxic, and safe to use when well-diluted and used in small amounts. You can use it for motion sickness and to aid digestion. It is very effective for pain relief caused by dysplasia, strains, arthritis, and sprains.

Helichrysum (Helichrysum italicum)

Well equipped with analgesic, anti-inflammatory, and regenerative properties, this essential oil is very therapeutic and thus excellent for skin irritations and skin conditions. You can also use it confidently on bruises and scars. It is great for relieving pain.

Lavender (Lavandula angustifolia)

Lavender is extremely gentle and safe. It has nerve-calming, anti-itch, and antibacterial properties. You can use it for numerous common ailments such as for first aid and for skin irritations.

Marjoram, Sweet (Origanum majorana)

If you want an essential oil that remedies bacterial skin infections, takes care of wounds, and repels insects at the same time, this is your oil. This essential oil is a calming muscle relaxant that has strong antibacterial properties.

Niaouli (Melaleuca Quinquenervia)

This oil has antihistaminic and powerful antibacterial properties. It is also more unlikely to cause irritation than tea tree. It is great for infections and irritation caused by allergies. This essential oil is Must-have oil for dog owners.

Peppermint (Mentha x piperita)

Peppermint is another one you should avoid if your dog is pregnant or small. The essential oil stimulates circulation and is antispasmodic. You can use it for strains and sprains, dysplasia, and arthritis. It is also a good insect repellant.

It works well with ginger to manage motion sickness.

Sweet Orange (Citrus sinensis)

This one is generally a deodorizing and calming essential oil that can also work as a flea-repellant.

Thyme ct. Linalool (Thymus vulgaris ct. linalool)

This essential oil is good for rheumatism, pain relief, and arthritis. It also has antibacterial, antiviral, and antifungal properties that make it excellent for infections and skin issues.

Valerian (Valeriana officinalis)

If your dog usually has a problem with anxiety issues such as noise anxiety and separation, you can use this nerve-calming essential oil.

How to Apply Essential Oils on Dogs

Here is how to use the above oils on your dog:

Aromatically

If you have a dog, you can use essential oils aromatically by dapping a drop of the essential oil on the dog bed or the collar. If you want to spray the dog's fur, add some essential oil drops to water and evenly spray the dog's fur.

NOTE: This method mainly targets to purify air, open airways, and manage moods.

Topically

If your dog is 15 lbs. or above, first dilute one drop of the essential oil to a tablespoon of fractionated coconut oil before you begin application.

If your dog is below this weight, dilute one drop of the essential oil to two tablespoons of fractionated coconut oil. For puppies, you can dilute one drop of the essential oil to 3 tablespoons of coconut oil.

If your dog is pregnant, sick, old, or prone to seizures, you should dilute one drop of the essential oil to three tablespoons of coconut oil.

You can also apply the essential oils to the pads/toes, spine, and ears of your dog. You can apply the essential oils directly to most areas of the dog's body but always avoid the nose, eyes, genital and anal areas.

Place some drops of the essential oil (preferably diluted) in your palms and rub them together then pet your dog.

Note: this method mainly:

1. Supports general health of the treated area

2. Provides immediate comfort

3. Supports the immune system

4. Supports the systemic health

Internally

This one aims to get the essential oil directly into the dog's body through ingestion. Therefore, add some drops to your dog's food or water then add some drops to a gelatin capsule and give to your dog.

This is particularly helpful if you want to:

1. Improve digestion

2. Improve oral health

3. Support health and throat comfort

4. Support liver health

NOTE: Before you let your dog ingest any essential oils, you should confirm that they are the best quality first. You can use 100% pure brands and those of therapeutic grade. In addition, administer only one drop when performing the application internally.

Additional Information

The veterinarian can also help you when you want to mix different essential oils to achieve a common objective. For instance,

Let us assume you want to improve your dog's ear health. Examples of essential oils that support great functioning of the ears include the following:

1. 5 drops of Lavender

2. 5 drops of Geranium

3. 5 drops of Melaleuca

You will mix all the ingredients in one tablespoon of coconut oil. Cleanse the ear using a natural cleaner, and then use a Q-tip (cotton-tipped swab usually used to cleanse a small section or during application of cosmetics or medications) to rub the mixture in the ear while making sure you do not push the Q-tip past where you cannot see it. Perform this two times a day until you see healthy skin.

If you want to support your dog's immune system for seasonal and environmental threats, you can do the following:

Place a drop of lemon, peppermint, and lavender in an empty capsule and either place it in food or give it directly to the dog. Since dogs are carnivorous, you need to make sure the diet is grain free: diet cause up to 95% of all food allergies in dogs. For this purpose, raw food or homemade diet is ideal.

Cats: Selecting Safe/The Best Essential Oils for Cats

This is where you need to pay keen attention. As mentioned earlier, cats are very sensitive to essential oils, which is why using essential oils with them is highly discouraged. Some cats have died after application of essential oils.

As you may already know, cats naturally lack glucuronidation, an important detox mechanism usually present in most animals. This simply means you have to be extra cautious if you are using any essential oils on your cat. Moreover, make sure to avoid everything you think may contain phenols so you avoid a build-up of toxic metabolites in your cat's body or worse, a possible fatal toxic shock.

For some time now, there have been reports about cats suffering from liver failure after exposure to essential oils such as using undiluted tea tree oil, or regular diffusion of different essential oils in a house. With that said, tea tree oil never makes an appearance on the list of safe essential oils for cats, even though it is widely used today.

Basic Guidelines for Using Essential Oils with Cats

1.   Let your cat decide. It is important to allow your cat a chance to choose if or not it wants a particular essential oil. If a cat resists an essential oil you have spent a fortune buying, do not force the oil on the cat: accept the loss☐.

2.   When the cat does not show any signs of rejecting the essential oil, dilute it well before application. You can use a drop in 25ml of carrier oil. We will discuss more on this shortly.

3.   It is not always prudent to put essential oils on your cat's body and even if you do not diffuse your essential oils frequently, never lock your cat in a room diffused with essential oils.

How to Know If Your Cat Wants/Needs a Particular Essential Oil

It is easy to know if your cat wants or needs a particular essential oil. Just hold the closed bottle in your hand not more than six inches away from your cat's nose. Patiently remain there for a while and allow the cat to come towards the bottle if he/she desires. Do not go towards the cat. Once you are sure your cat likes the essential oil, you can go ahead and dilute the essential oil and apply it on the cat.

In case you are wondering, these are the signs of interest you should expect: the cat sniffs the bottle, makes a brief sniff, goes but returns to the bottle, his/her tongue licks quickly, and is distracted from the aromas easily.

If your cat turns away from the aroma and leaves the room, you should take this as a sign of disinterest. In this case, do not apply.

NOTE: You should also remember that since cats are extremely sensitive to essential oils, a couple of sniffs are enough to stimulate the healing process. Again, cats are quite subtle—actually more than dogs in their response to essential oils—and you may find them annoyingly secretive if you are not keen enough.

Thus, if the cat stays with you in the room when the bottle is open, count it as a positive response even if the cats shows signs of feeling otherwise or acting indifferent or nonchalant. If you notice the cat showing signs of wanting to lick the oil (which is very rare), you can allow it to lick only a few drops of diluted oil from your fingers if possible, or pour a few drops on a saucer and leave it on the floor, far from the cat's usual eating area.

Many experienced essential oils users will tell you that cats rarely get comfortable with application of essential oils on their skin. Thus, expect to stick to a few little sniffs (inhalation method of application) to bring about a strong change even if you want to treat wounds.

Selecting Safe/The Best Essential Oils for Cats

With that said, we will discuss essential oils that are safe, acceptable, and effective to use with cats.

Myrrh

Owing to its powerful cleansing properties, Myrrh is particularly good for the throat and mouth; it is soothing to the skin and great in terms of supporting emotional balance and awareness. You should use it to maintain peaceful feelings when tension levels are peaking in your cat.

Lavender

This essential oil offers cats relaxing feelings and calmness. It soothes occasional irritation on the skin and eases tense feelings, reduces anxious feelings, and supports restful/better sleep.

Frankincense

For a healthy cellular function, frankincense should be your choice. It also brings about relaxation, mood balance, rejuvenates the skin, and soothes the entire body.

Helichrysum

This essential oil is particularly useful in promoting healthy metabolism, soothing the skin, and promoting vitality and energy.

Digestive blend

This is a blend of oils such as aloe juice, coconut oil, cod liver oil, cedar wood oil, lavender oil that promote good digestions. Today, there are digestive blend essential oils retailed, which means you do not have to blend the essential oils yourself. This is a good example.

Digestive blend oils are great for road trips. They support a healthy digestion and soothe stomach discomfort, improve the gastrointestinal tract, help relieve feelings of queasiness, reduce bloating, and occasional indigestion and gas.

Grounding blend

Just like the digestive blend, the grounding essential oil is good for emotional relaxation. This blend is a combination of seven therapeutic grade oils that include:

1. Ylang Ylang Essential Oil (Cananga odorata)

2. Spruce Essential Oil (Picea mariana)

3. Cedarwood Essential Oil (Cedras atlantica)

4. Juniper Essential Oil (Juniperus osteosperma)

5. White Fir Essential Oil (Abies concolor)

6. Pine Essential Oil (Pinus sylvestris)

7. Angelica Essential Oil (Angelica archangelica)

This essential oil supports a complete sense of relaxation, stimulates feelings of tranquility, balance, and eases feelings of anxiety. You should use it in car rides to stimulate feelings of calmness.

Protective blend

An essential oil blend that offers protection is also a good alternative to the numerous synthetic options offered out there for immune support. By using these oils, it enhances your cat's natural body antioxidant defenses. In the end, you protect your feline friend against seasonal and environmental threats, and encourage a healthy respiratory function.

Juniper Berry

This essential oil is also good for a healthy urinary tract and kidney function. Apart from being a natural skin toner, it also acts as a natural detoxifying and cleansing agent for cats, which you can use as part of a natural cleansing regimen. If you decide to use it, remember to combine it with cypress: they blend very well.

Arborvitae

Arborvitae is a versatile essential oil that acts as a natural insect repellant, protects against seasonal and environmental threats, acts as a strong cleansing and purifying agent, grounding aroma, and induces feelings of calmness and peace. This one naturally blends perfectly with frankincense and cedarwood.

Other effective essential oils

1. Bergamot

2. Clementine

3. Eucalyptus

4. Frankincense

5. Juniper

6. Lavandin

7. Lime

8. Orange (Bitter, Blood, Sweet)

9. Peppermint

10. Rosemary

11. Spearmint

12. Tangerine

13. Yarrow

14. Camphor

15. Clove (Bud, Leaf, Stem)

16. Fir

17. Grapefruit

18. Lemon

19. Mandarin

20. Oregano

21. Pine

22. Sage

23. Spruce

24. Thyme

Basic Essential Oil Application Guidelines For Cats

When it comes to cats, you can use various ways to apply essential oils. Of all these methods, water diffusion is the best. You can also use 4 drops of essential oil and one cup of baking soda to create a litter box powder with essential oils. Stir well and let it sit for 12 hours to saturate the baking soda with the essential oil. Sprinkle the mixture on your cat's litter (a bit of it, enough to cover the litter, not the entire cup).

You can also apply the oils topically, a process that requires dilution using the recommended ratio we mentioned earlier. Once you dilute the oils, you can then use the easiest way to apply the essential oils topically on cats, which is by petting along the spine.

Another way is using the reflexology points or rubbing the tips of the ears if your cat can agree to such applications. Simply place one drop of the essential oil in your hand and swirl it clockwise with the other hand; use your finger to apply on your cat. To dilute, you can add a drop of a carrier oil such as organic olive. It is good to use therapeutic grade essential oils because they absorb well and rarely build up. In any case, when you notice an irritation developing, you can also use the carrier oil for dilution; this is, however, a very rare occurrence.

The cat will consume the essential oils through grooming when you use topical application and that is mainly the reason why dilution is important.

CAUTION: Like in humans, avoid dropping oils in the cat's eyes or ears. If you are not sure about how to do the best application on the ear, you can place a drop of oil on one palm of your hand and use a finger from your other hand to apply the oil on the inside of the upper part of the ear.

For internal application, you have to be more careful. Begin with a toothpick drop of the essential oil and mix it with the food—the food should be wet. You, however, have to note that some cats get very fussy when it comes to food, and will refuse the food if it contains oil; others do not mind it at all. You have to be very observant. Your observations of your cat's behavior will tell you what works best for him/her.

BONUS: Additional Information

When buying essential oils for all pets:

1.   Look for essential oils bottled either in cobalt, amber, or violet glass bottles.

2.   Search for essential information of the oils: check the label, the brochure, or the store's website information, etc. This is what you should look for:

•   The oil's common name; for instance, Lavender

•   The oil's Latin name; for instance, Lavandula angustifolia

•   The country of origin

•   The oil extraction process

•   The term '100% pure essential oil'

•   Cultivation method-for instance, organic, wildharvested, cultivated etc

The information you get on the points above should make sense (on the particular brand you want to purchase), and correspond to what many sources (such as the internet, your vet, and this book) say about the brand.

3.   Essential oils are usually expensive; it is not prudent to go for ridiculously cheap oils because such oils are more likely to be adulterated.

Conclusion

We have come to the end of the book. Thank you for reading and congratulations for reading until the end.

What you have just read is the ultimate guide to natural essential oils for pets. Now that you have the basic and most important knowledge about selecting the right essential oils, the ideal application procedure, and the precautions that come with it, you are ready to use essential oils to transform, protect, and maintain your pet accordingly.

If you found the book valuable, can you recommend it to others? One way to do that is to post a review on Amazon.

Please leave a review for this book on Amazon!

Thank you and good luck!

Preview Of 'Anti-Inflammatory Diet Guide

,

Effects Of Inflammation

Inflammation is the biological response your body goes into when dealing with harmful stimuli such as irritants, pathogens or even damaged cells. It is a self-protection mechanism that allows your body to begin the healing process. The 'hotness' or 'inflammation' you feel after you cut yourself or injure yourself is the result of your body working hard to heal itself. But what happens when your body experiences 'too much' inflammation?

A little inflammation is not a bad thing. In fact, when it happens, you should rejoice in knowing that your body is working tirelessly to correct the situation. However, like most good things, inflammation can get out of hand. When this happens, you may experience various health complications such as:

Weight Gain

Every day, thousands of people try to lose weight to no avail. They complain that they've tried out various diets but somehow none seem to be working. If they do find something that works, sooner than later, they are back to gaining the weight they thought they'd lost. This is because they neglect to look into inflammation as the cause for their weight gain. Inflammation contributes to weight gain in various ways. These include:

• If inflammation happens in the brain, it interferes with the functioning of the hypothalamus and this in turn increases your appetite and slows down your metabolism. When this happens, you will be eating a lot but burning up less energy, which leads to weight gain.

• Gut inflammation leads to leptin and insulin resistance. Leptin is the satiety hormone that tells your brain when you have had enough. When suffering from leptin resistance, you just eat and eat some more before leptin can communicate that you have had enough, which leads to weight gain. Another thing that gut inflammation does is to increase intestinal permeability. When this happens, more toxins will be able to permeate your bloodstream. Usually toxins are stored in fat cells to remove them from circulation. The more toxins you have, the more the fat cells expand to accommodate the more toxins leading to weight gain.

• Inflammation in the endocrine system suppresses adrenal and thyroid function. One of the main functions of the adrenal gland is to burn fat. Therefore, when you suppress the functioning of the adrenal gland, you are unable to burn fat, as you should leading to weight gain.

As you have read, inflammation is bad for you if you want to maintain the ideal weight.

Metabolic Syndrome

Metabolic syndrome refers to a group/cluster of lifestyle-related diseases including cardiovascular disease and obesity. They are clustered together because all of these diseases are linked to metabolic dysfunction. Markers of metabolic dysfunction include:

• Central obesity – this is excessive tummy fat

• Hyperinsulinaemia – this refers to ongoing high levels of insulin

• Insulin resistance –your body loses sensitivity to insulin (you need more insulin to manage your blood sugar levels)

But the question is how these three factors are connected. Well, when on a diet high in carbohydrates, your blood sugar levels increase leading to high insulin levels to help blood cells absorb the glucose and thus manage your blood sugar levels. When you have high insulin levels, the production of cytokines (which are pro-inflammatory) increases and in turn this causes inflammation especially in predisposed persons. Once inflammation increases, it brings with it an increase in the production of free radicals. Free radicals affect cellular functions and one of those functions just happens to be insulin sensitivity. This is why chroni low-grade inflammation is linked to all three markers; that is, raised insulin levels, obesity and decreased insulin sensitivity.

Chronic Fatigue

Many people suffering from chronic fatigue have been told that the disease 'is all in their minds'. Fortunately, in recent years more researchers have began looking into the association of chronic fatigue and inflammation. This is mainly because the two possess many similar symptoms including muscular pain and tenderness, sore throat, joint pain, swollen lymph nodes and sore throat.

As you know, inflammation is the way your body reacts to foreign particles. When you have symptoms of inflammation, it is safe to say that your body is fighting something even if that something is not yet known. This is why researchers link an overactive immune system to chronic fatigue.

Another thing that associates chronic fatigue with inflammation is the lack of cortisol in patients suffering from chronic fatigue. Cortisol is known to suppress inflammation. Thus, if your body has a cortisol deficiency, it will not be able to suppress inflammation and this will worsen symptoms of chronic fatigue. A dietary change often helps people suffering from chronic fatigue.

Some types of arthritis

When you hear the name arthritis, you automatically associate it with pain. Well, it is no coincidence since arthritis refers to inflammation in joints. When your joints experience inflammation, you will feel pain. The types of arthritis that have been linked to inflammation include:

- Gouty arthritis

- Rheumatoid arthritis

- Psoriatic arthritis

- Systematic lupus erythematosus

When you suffer from these types of arthritis, you may experience inflammation symptoms such as redness, joint stiffness, swelling of the joints, pain in the joints and loss of joint function.

It is important to note that inflammation does not have to be painful for it to be present. This is because many organs in your body just don't have enough pain-sensitive areas for you to feel that inflammatory sensation. This means that you can suffer from chronic inflammation over time without knowing, only for you to experience the effects of inflammation.

It is also important to note that various things can cause inflammation including:

- Processed foods high in sugar and unhealthy fats

- Omega-6 fats (and not enough Omega-3 fatty acids)

- Sleep deprivation

- Chronic stress

- Smoking

- Pollution

- Environmental chemicals

- Lack of exercise

Thus, chances are, if you experience any of the above things, you may be suffering from inflammation whether or not you experience pain.

The first thing you should do once you notice that you suffer from inflammation is not to reach for drugs because drugs just address the symptoms and not the root cause but rather to make some lifestyle changes. This is because most of the causes of inflammation can be addressed by making lifestyle changes like exercising more, reducing exposure to pollutants, not smoking and dietary changes.

In this book, we will focus on addressing inflammation by adopting an anti-inflammatory diet. Let us learn more about anti-inflammatory diet in the next chapter.

Check out the rest of Anti-Inflammatory Diet Guide on Amazon.

Or go to: **http://amzn.to/2qKTSPa**

Check Out My Other Books

Below you'll find some of my other popular books on Amazon and Kindle as well. Simply search for the title on the Amazon website to find it.

Belly Diet: The Zero Belly Diet Step-By-Step Guide Which Help You To Lose Your Belly And Enjoy Your Flat Belly

Anti-Inflammatory Diet Guide: The Guide To Reduce Inflammation And Live A Healthy Life Without Pain

Negative Calorie Diet: Cookbook & Guide Which Will Help You To Burn Body Fat, Lose Weight And Live Healthy

Clean Eating: Cookbook And Guide To Restore Your Body's Natural Balance And Eat Healthy

Dash Diet: Cookbook For Weight Loss With Action Plan And Easy Recipes

Freedom: How To Make Money Online And Become Financially Free By Creating Passive Income

Weight Loss: 20 Easy And Fast Diet Tips For Losing Weight – An Easy-To-Follow Weight Loss Guide

Smart Fat: Cookbook With Fat Meals Which Help You To Lose Weight, Get Healthy And Improve Brain Function

Habits Of Highly Effective People: What are the habits of successful people?

78209209R00027

Made in the USA
Columbia, SC
04 October 2017